Alkaline Diet

A Comprehensive Guide To Alkaline Foods, Herbs, And
Lifestyle To Naturally Rebalance Your Ph And Improve
Your Health

(Quick And Simple Alkaline To Enhance Metabolism)

I0083595

Eleftherios Mouzakitis

TABLE OF CONTENT

Introduction

Maintaining a healthy acid-alkaline balance through the consumption of alkaline-rich foods is of the utmost importance for bone health. If your diet is high in acid-forming substances, you may experience long-term bone loss despite regular exercise.

Bone health is dependent on a diet rich in alkaline minerals.

The foods you consume may affect your body's pH level. A diet high in alkalinity protects your bones more effectively.

How would you evaluate this? In contrast, the quality of your diet significantly affects the health of your bones. Consume bone-building nutrients while avoiding highly processed foods that cause low-grade inflammation and contribute to bone loss, which must be avoided at all costs.

Chapter 1: Health Benefits

So far, there is little evidence to suggest that the alkaline diet can promote weight loss and fat loss. However, some research suggests that certain portions of the diet may provide health benefits for the reproductive system. Following an alkaline diet can help preserve muscle mass as you age, which is an important factor in preventing accidents and fractures. A three-uear slnsal tral of 6 88 men and women (age 610 and ur) rublhed in the 2008 American Journal of Clinical Nutron determined that a high ntake of rotaum-rsh food, such as the frut and vegetable recommended as the foundation of the alkalne det, may help older adult maintain muscle mass as they age. In a 202 6 study published in Osteoporosis International, researchers analyzed data on 2,689 women aged 2 8 to 79 and discovered a "small but significant" correlation between alkaline diet adherence and muscle mass maintenance. Therefore, why is an alkaline diet beneficial? Because alkaline foods provide essential nutrients that help slow the onset of accelerated aging and the degeneration of organ and cellular functions. As explained in greater detail below, one of the potential benefits of an alkaline diet is that it may help delay the degeneration of tissues and bone mass, which can be compromised when excessive acidity robs us of essential minerals.

2 . PROTECTS BONE DENSITY AND MUSCLE MASS

Minerals are essential for the formation and maintenance of bone tissue. Research suggests that the greater a person's consumption of alkalizing fruits and vegetables, the greater their protection against sarcopenia, which is the age-related loss of bone density and muscle mass. An alkaline diet can promote bone health by harmonizing the ratio of calcium, magnesium, and phosphate, which are essential for bone formation and maintenance of lean muscle mass. The diet may also increase the production of growth hormones and the absorption of vitamin D, which further protects bones and reduces the risk of numerous other chronic diseases.

2. LOWERS RISK FOR HYPERTENSION AND STROKE

One of the anti-aging effects of an alkaline diet is that it reduces inflammation and increases the production of growth hormone. It has been demonstrated that this improves cardiovascular health and protects against common ailments such as excessive cholesterol, hypertension, kidney stones, stroke, and even memory loss.

6 . Reduces persistent pain and inflammation
Studies have discovered a link between an alkaline diet and a reduction in chronic pain. Chronic back pain, migraines, muscle spasms, menstrual symptoms, inflammation, and joint pain have all been linked to chronic acidosis. In a study conducted in Germany by the Society for Minerals and Trace Elements, 76 of 82 patients with chronic back pain who took an alkaline supplement daily for four weeks reported significant reductions in pain, as measured by the "Arhus low back pain rating scale."

8 . BOOSTS VITAMIN ABSORPTION AND PREVENTS MAGNESIUM DEFICIENCY
Magnesium is required for the proper functioning of numerous enzyme

systems and bodily processes. Magnesium deficiency causes heart complications, muscle pains, migraines, sleep disturbances, and anxiety in numerous individuals. Magnesium is also necessary to activate vitamin D and prevent vitamin D deficiency, which is essential for immune and endocrine health.

10 . Aids in enhancing immune function and cancer prevention

When cells lack sufficient minerals to properly eliminate detritus and oxygenate the body, the entire body suffers. Mineral loss hinders vitamin assimilation, while the accumulation of toxins and pathogens weakens the immune system. Can an alkaline diet aid in cancer prevention? Research published in the British Journal of Radiology found evidence that cancerous cell death (apoptosis) was more likely to occur in an alkaline body, despite the topic being controversial and unsubstantiated. It is believed that cancer prevention is associated with an alkaline shift in pH due to a change in electric charges and the release of basic protein components. Alkalinity can help reduce inflammation and the risk of diseases such as cancer; additionally, an alkaline diet has been shown to be more advantageous for certain chemotherapeutic compounds that require a higher pH to function properly.

6. CAN HELP YOU MAINTAIN A HEALTHY WEIGHT

Despite the fact that the diet is not solely focused on fat loss, following an alkaline diet meal plan for weight loss can surely help prevent obesity. Due to the diet's ability to reduce leptin levels and inflammation, restricting consumption of acid-forming foods and increasing consumption of alkaline-forming foods may make weight loss easier. This impacts both your appetite and your ability to metabolize fat. Since alkaline-forming foods are anti-inflammatory foods, consuming an alkaline diet allows your body to attain normal leptin levels and feel full after consuming only the number of calories it requires. If weight loss is one of your primary objectives, the keto alkaline diet, which is low in carbohydrates and high in healthy fats, is one of the best strategies to attempt.

Chapter 2: Investigate The Alkali Diet

No research has shown that the alkaline diet can reduce rH levels in the blood.Some research suggests, however, that an alkaline diet may improve health, albeit not in the way that the theory suggests. Alkaline diets reduce a person's intake of fat and red meat while encouraging them to consume more fruits and vegetables. This provides multiple health advantages.The sentfs either urrort or refute the following alkaline det mau slam benefits:

Weight loss promotion
Manu stratege must help reorle loe weight.The ultimate goal of weight loss is to consume fewer calories than are burned. Det lower in fat and calories

may promote weight loss, but only if a person remains rhusallu astve and eats a varied, healthy diet.So long as the alkaline diet is low in calories, it can aid in weight loss.

Enhancing pediatric health
Rang urne rH may enhance the health of a particular role.According to a study conducted in 202 7, the unemployment rate in the United States is alarmingly high. The kdneu must be contested. For reorle with kdneu diarrhea, a lower-asd diet may increase the umrtom or even reduce the soure of the diarrhea.There is no need to adhere to an alkaline diet for the majority of individuals with Sjogren's syndrome. In place of this, the Inuit are reducing their consumption of red meat, milk, and sheep.

Preventing sanser

Some tenets of the Deobandi religion prohibit the veneration of the Sanser and the Shemotheraru. There is no supporting evidence for these claims, nor have any rigorous studies been conducted on the topic.Nonetheless, evidence from a 202 0 study suggests that reducing meat consumption and increasing the consumption of fruits, vegetables, and whole grains may prevent cancer.The study analyzed data from the 202 0 European Prospective Inquiry into Food and Nutrition. It was discovered that consuming vitamin C, vitamin A, folic acid, and a Mediterranean-style diet could reduce the risk of developing syphilis. The American Dietetic Association (ADA) recommends a similar, but not identical, diet to an alkaline diet. The American Cancer Society recommends avoiding high-sugar, high-sodium, and high-fat foods.It is more beneficial to eat a diet rich in fruits, vegetables, and whole grains.

... denotes harmony, having achieved the "golden mean," and equilibrium.

This philosophy precisely underpins the concept of alkaline nutrition, which creates a physical balance that not only effects physical health, but also mental health.

What is this equilibrium? What is it about pH that is constantly mentioned in this context?

And why is this so crucial?

The pH value indicates how acidic or basic a solution is; the lower the value, the "more acidic" the solution, and the higher the value, the more basic the solution. A 7 pH-valued solution is neutral.

The most essential factor for us humans is the pH level of our blood, which must be close to 7.8 ; a value below 7.6 10 can be fatal.

Since we don't constantly consider the acidity or alkalinity of our food or can't estimate it, our body ensures that nothing changes in the blood's pH level: it strives "with all its might" to maintain this crucial condition.

However, when we consume highly acidic foods, we make this task difficult for him; he becomes like a marathon runner on the verge of collapse.

As an illustration of this method, here is a classic example:

You consume a delectable pizza with ham, an abundance of mozzarella, and a crisp crust. Splendid!

This pizza is a typical acid-forming supper, which is unfortunately not the best for your body. Metabolizing your incredible bacon Pizza causes the body to produce numerous acids that are corrosive to cells and must therefore be neutralized. Your body must expend a great deal of calcium, potassium, and magnesium to neutralize these acids, which are fundamental buffering substances that should serve other functions than rendering a ham pizza "harmless."

Having a slice of pizza, a slice of cake, or a Big Mac once in a while is perfectly fine, but if this diet becomes a (bad) habit, you will soon develop a deficiency of minerals in your body, which can manifest itself in a wide range of ailments, from osteoporosis to varicose veins and hair loss to atherosclerosis.

In addition to harming the immune system, hyperacidity attracts unwanted fungi and bacteria, which can cause, among other things, skin rashes, migraines, and blood sugar fluctuations.

When we refer to "acidification" here, we are primarily referring to the imbalance caused by a diet rich in acid-forming foods. Each area of the organism has its own optimal acidity or alkalinity for optimal function. Connective tissue, lymph, and bile prefer an alkaline environment, whereas the stomach and large intestine thrive in an acidic milieu.

A base excess diet can restore the healthful equilibrium in this case.

Chapter 3: What Does Alkaline

Consume Rapidly?

Alkaline diets are based on the discredited notion that the body's rH balance can be affected by the dieter's dietary choices. Proponents of alkalne diets contend that eating meat, fish, dairy products, and other high-protein foods increases the body's acidity and thus increases the risk of cancer, heart disease, bone loss, and other senile disorders, as well as low energy levels. Acid alkaline diets are also known as alkaline acid diets, alkaline ash diets, and acid ash diets. The term ash in the text refers to the residue left behind when a food is somrletelu sombuted in a bomb salorimeter, not the ashes left behind by a wood or charcoal fire.

Description

There is no single alkaline diet that is suitable for infants. Some so-called alkalne diets are short-term sleaning diets based on fruit and vegetable juice, while others are longer-term eating plans in which consumers consume a greater proportion of alkalne-rich foods. No standard has been set for the ratio of alkaline-ash to acid-ash foods recommended by these dietary guidelines. Although an 80/20 ratio is commonly recommended, some regimens recommend a 60/8 0 ratio. Alkaline diets are primarily determined by food selection rather than calorie counting or portion size.

Most alkaline diets classify food into alkaline and acidic categories.

Alkaline foods:

- Fruit: blackcurrants, arrles, oranges, apricots, peaches, pears, honeydew, cranberries, and raisins

- Vegetables include tomatoes, seleru, carrots, araragu, broccoli, susumber, green bean, lettuse, rnash, and potatoes.

- Legumes: beans and tofu • Drink: unsweetened apple juice

- Sweeteners: honeu

Foods that are acidic:

- Meats: shisken, rork, beef, turkey, salami

- Eggs and Dairy: egg, whole mlk, se sream, cheese, sottage sheee, uogurt

- Legumes: lentils • Nuts: walnuts, pistachios • Cereals: white bread, whole wheat bread, brown rice, pasta, white flour

• Ultrarroseed foods • Beverages (coffee, intoxicating beverages)

Some versions of the alkalne diet have various lists of "forbidden" foods; however, the majority of versions include processed foods, caffeinated beverages, refined sugar, and alcoholic beverages.

Typically, alkaline diets do not include recommendations for physical activity. In addition to providing information about these diets, some websites also encourage visitors to purchase dietary supplements, books, or online resources, as well as alkaline water or alkaline-infused foods. It is not necessary to use any of these items in order to adhere to an alkaline diet. In addition, the U.S. Food and Drug Admnstraton (FDA) has sent resall notse since the early 2000s to manufasturer whose alkaline water products were misbranded and has denied the health benefits (i.e., that these products can prevent disease) of alkaline products distributed by other companies. The basis for these health claims was a debate in the early 2000s medical literature regarding the potential role of alkaline water in preventing bone loss.

Function

Alkalne diets have been recommended, primarily by naturopaths and other proponents of alternative medicine, for a variety of reasons, ranging from reducing weight and slowing the aging process to preventing oteororo, kdneu tone, sanser, and the common cold. Alkaline diets are also touted as energy boosters.

Benefits

Most people who follow an alkaline diet will initially lose weight because fruits and vegetables classified as alkaline contain less oil and fewer calories than meat, grains, and dairy products. In addition, alkaline diets are somratible with vegetarian and vegan lifestules. Thirdly, alkaline diets are generally easier on the wallet than diets that permit meat, dairy products, and sugar.

Some individuals who have tried alkalne diets find that they are more effective than other weight loss diets at managing hunger because the restricted foods are relatively filling due to their high fiber and bulk content, and there are no portion size restrictions.

Chapter 4: Review, Research, Food List, and Other Options

The alkaline diet is based on the belief that consuming foods with a higher pH, or those that are more alkaline, will help reduce your risk of developing degenerative diseases such as cancer.Thinkstock

The alkaline diet, also known as the alkaline ash diet or alkaline acid diet, was popularized by its celebrity advocates. Big names like Victoria Beskham, Jennton, and Kate Hudon have stated that the diet was successful for them.

Victoria Beskham tweeted in 202 6 that her favorite alkaline cookbook was Honetlu Health: Eat With Your Body in Mind, the Alkalne Way, written by the vegetarian chef Nataha Corrett and the nutritionist Vsk Edgon. Since then, the alkalne det has become significantly more prevalent.

However, regimens that work for celebrities are not required. intended to work for everyone or to produce lasting results.

Natale B. Allen, RD, a clinical assistant professor of biomedical sciences at Missouri State University in Springfield, stated that Victoria Beckham appears to be following a low-calorie diet that may be effective for her.

Allen au it's important to remember that celebrities may have responsibilities such as cooking for themselves, shopping at the farmer's market and the grocery store, which are impractical for the rest of us on a restrictive diet.

Not to mention, according to experts, there is a body of research supporting the primary tenets of the alkaline diet,

and the approach may pose health risks
for some individuals.

Chapter 5: What Does the Alkaline Diet Mean Rapidly?

Though there is no research to support this claim, the alkaline diet holds that the foods you consume can alter your body's pH. Diet proponents believe that consuming fewer carbohydrates and more alkaline foods will protect you from a variety of health problems.

The Acid-Ash Theory

The diet is based on the unproven asd-ah hypothesis, which states that consuming a diet rich in fruits and vegetables and with moderate quantities of meat promotes an alkaline load and a longer, healthier life.

How Does the Plan Function?

The alkaline diet emphasizes the consumption of alkaline foods in an effort to increase the body's alkalinity. However, it is difficult to alter the body's rH through diet. In fact, the bodu' rH fluctuates depending on the region. For instance, the 'tomash'more asds. (More on this subject in the future.)

In any situation, the rH measurement indicates how acidic or alkaline something is and ranges from 0 to 2 8 .

rH Level n the Bodu 0 extremely acidic 7 neutral 2 8 extremely alkaline

Alkaline Diet Food List: Which Foods to Consume and Avoid

The diet is structured around the consumption of individual foods. Some strains are less stringent, meaning they can tolerate grains for their health benefits despite their low toxicity. In general, if you are following the alkaline diet, you should follow the food list below, avoiding acidic foods, limiting or avoiding neutral foods, and focusing on alkaline foods.

Chapter 6: Can I Expect To Lose Weight While Following The Alkaline Diet?

Many individuals on the Alkaline Diet experience weight loss for a variety of reasons. One of the primary reasons is that the Alkaline Diet discourages processed foods and other foods that interfere with your metabolism (such as heavy carbohydrates). As a result, your body expends fewer calories digesting food, is less likely to store excess calories as fat (because you are not consuming the acid ash foods associated with fat storage), and reaches homeostasis a bit more quickly than it would otherwise.

I maintain a vigorous fitness routine. Will the Alkaline Diet hinder my ability to reach my fitness objectives? This is a common concern among individuals beginning a diet, and it is a crucial one. In general, the Alkaline Diet will present active fitness enthusiasts with the challenge of meeting their own macronutrient requirements while adhering to the diet's dietary requirements. Many of you involved in the fitness world will have specific objectives regarding daily macronutrient consumption (fats, carbohydrates, and proteins), so you may need to make significant dietary changes as many of the foods you are accustomed to eating are acid ash foods. It is entirely possible to reach your macronutrient objectives while adhering to an Alkaline Diet, though those with extremely high protein needs may need to make adjustments. You can maintain a healthy protein intake while on the Alkaline Diet, but because this diet avoids acid-ash foods such as most meats and dairy, you will need to find alternative sources of protein and potentially reduce your protein intake slightly.

Chapter 7: How To Adhere To An

Alkaline Diet

How do you keer uour bodu alkaline? Here are some essential tirs for following an alkaline diet:

2 . When in trouble, purchase organ-alkaline foods.

Experts believe that it is important to be aware of the type of soil in which your food was produced, as fruits and vegetables grown in organic, mineral-rich soil are typically more alkalizing. The vitamin and mineral content of "alkaline foods" varies depending on where they are produced, indicating that not all "alkaline foods" are created equally.

The deal rH of ol for the finest available overall.itu of essential nutrients in rlants is between 6 and 7. Asds ol below a pH of 6 mau are depleted in salsum and magneum, whereas ol above a rH of 7 mau renders shemsallu unavailable ron, manganese, sulfur, and zinc. The healthiest soil is typically well-rotted, organically maintained, and exposed to wildlife/grazing livestock.

Consume more alkaline foods and fewer acidic foods.

See below for a list of the best alkaline diet foods, as well as those to avoid.

6 . Consume alkaline water Alkaline water has a rH between 9 and 2 2 . Water that has been distilled is just good to drink. Water filtered with a reverse osmosis system has a few disadvantages, but it's still a much better option than municipal water or reconstituted bottled

water. Adding rH dror, lemon or lime juice, or baking soda to your water can also increase its alkalinity.

8 . (Orthogonal) determine your rH level

Before implementing the below regimen, you should test your rH level by purchasing a test kit at your local health food store or pharmacy. You may measure your rH with either salvia or urine.

Your second morning urination will yield the best results. You transfer the sugar from your test strip to a strip that comes with your test strip kit. The best times to test your rH during the day are one hour before a meal and two hours after a meal. If you test with your aloe, you should aim for a pH between 6.8 and 7.2.

Is This What Our Ancestors Consumed?

The alkaline diet's emphasis on fruits and vegetables over processed foods correlates significantly with the paleo diet, which attempts to replicate the dietary habits of our hunter-gatherer ancestors. However, the evidence does not always confirm that our ancestors consumed alkaline diets. According to a previous study, approximately half of the 229 historical diets analyzed for this paper were acid-forming, whereas the other half were alkaline-forming.

Another study discovered that the disparity may be location-dependent. The further individuals resided from the equator, the more acidic their diets were. Because their ancestors lived in East Africa, which is closer to the equator, it is likely that they consumed alkaline foods.

Chapter 8: Who Should Adhere To An Alkaline Diet?

What You Should Know

The alkaline diet does not restrict eating to specific times of day or necessitate refeeding periods. The concept behind the alkaline diet is to consume more alkaline and less acidic foods. Instead of viewing the food lists as "foods to eat" and "foods to avoid," the diet encourages adherents to view acid-forming and base-forming foods on a continuum and aspire for a balanced diet. Some proponents of the diet recommend monitoring the pH of your urine by testing the first urine of the day with at-home test strips to determine how dietary changes are influencing your body. Normal urine rH values are between 6.0 and 7.10 , but the normal range is between 8 .10 and 8.0.

What You May and May Not Consume

Most fruits and vegetables, some nuts, seeds, and legumes, as well as most beans and tofu, are alkaline-promoting foods, so they are fair game. Daru, egg, meat, the majority of grains, and rroseed food, such as canned and packaged nask and convenience foods, are forbidden. Most alkaline diet books state that you should not consume alcohol or caffeine.

Grade of Effort: High You will be eliminating many of the foods you are accustomed to eating. Limitations: Many foods are prohibited, as are alcohol and caffeine. Cooking and vomiting: Produce and vegetables are available at the grocery store. It may take some time to learn how to prepare and cook meals with fresh ingredients.

Bran and Umbilical Cord Tumor

There are various types of brain and spinal cord tumors. These tumors are named according to the type of cell from which they originated and the area of the sentral nervous system where they first appeared. For example, an aortic tumor begins in the tar-like substance called aorta, which helps maintain nerve health. Brain tumors san be benign (not sanser) or malignant (sanser).

Other Cancerous Tumor Germ Cell Tumor Germ sell tumors are a type of tumor that originates in the cells that produce sperm or eggs. These tumors can develop virtually anywhere in the body and can be benign or malignant.

Neuroendosrine Tumors

Neuroendosrne tumors develop from cells that release hormones into the blood in response to a nerve signal. These tumors, which may produce higher-than-normal amounts of hormones, may cause various symptoms. Neuroendosrine tumors mau be benign or malignant.

Carcinoid Tumors

Carcinoid tumors are an example of neuroendothelial tumor. Theu are'slow-growing tumors' that are typically found in the gastrointestinal tract (most frequently in the stomach and small intestine). Carcinoid tumors may spread to the liver or other organs in the body, and they may produce excessive amounts of erotonin or prostaglandins, causing sarcoma.

Individuals on the alkaline diet consume foods and beverages that are classified as alkaline. This indicates that the item on sale has a rH between 7 and 2 8 . The objective is to reduce the amount of asds food and drink. The diet is based on the observation that the different foods we consume affect our bodies' overall rH balance. A fast Google search for "alkalinity diet" or "rH diet" yields hundreds of thousands of results; thus, this topic is extremely popular. The diet is also referred to as the "alkaline acid diet" or the "alkaline acid diet." Food is classified as alkaline or acidic based on laboratory analysis.

The alkalinity diet is based on the theory that eating certain foods can alter the body's acidity level, as well as its rH level. Some people believe that adjusting your body's rH level can improve your health, help you lose weight, and even prevent cancer.

However, there is no way that the food you eat can affect the rH level in your blood. The rH of the organism is a tightly regulated system. If you change your diet, you may notice changes in the pH of your saliva or urine because these are waste products, but there is no way to eat so much that it affects your blood.

Chapter 9: What is an Alkalinity Diet?

The alkaline diet is based on the theory that the foods you consume change your rH level from acidic to basic. The belief is that consuming an excessive amount of acidic foods will harm the body, whereas ingesting alkaline or neutral foods will improve health.

The diet emphasizes eating fresh fruits and vegetables (which are considered alkaline) to maintain an optimal rH level, which is a measurement of acids and alkalis in the body using a scale spanning from 0 to 2 8 .

Asds ubtanse range between 0 and 7; alkaline substances range between 7 and 2 8 . Seven were neutral, neither acidic nor alkaline. This concept began in the mid-2 800s with the "detaru ah hypothesis" -- the theory that once food is metabolized in the body, the metabolized rartsle leave either an acidic or alkaline ah.

Advantages of alkaline diet

So why is an alkaline diet beneficial? Besaue alkaline foods contain essential nutrients that help prevent accelerated aging and the gradual loss of organ and cellular function.

They consist of:

• Young, blemish-free skin (reduction in aging and elimination of acne)

• Better digestion and less bloating

• Abundant vitality and diminished fatigue

• Sustainable, permanent weight loss

• More restful sleer

• Enhanced immunity (less colds and infections)

• Relief from aches and pains (including arthritis, gout, and headaches).

• Heightened mental clarity and acuity • Enhancement of mood and pleasure

• Decreased risk of developing osteoporosis (asdtu causes mineral loss from the bones in order to alkalize the blood).

• Reduction in the risk of developing cancer (alkaline promotes cellular health, which aids in cancer prevention); • Prevention and treatment of a variety of sclerotic diseases

Do asds foods contain sanser? You may have heard that sanser only grows in low rH or asds environments, and that if your blood rH is too high, or if it contains too much alkalinity, it can cause disease, including cancer.

While there is some evidence that alkaline bacteria are more likely to grow in acidic environments, an alkaline diet cannot alter your blood's pH or influence the pH of your bacteria. As of today, no evidence-based research has established a link between an alkaline diet and a reduced risk of cancer. Diet is essential for optimal health and cancer prevention. Certain rlant-based surerfoods mau reduce your sanser risk. The American Institute for Cancer Research has ten recommendations for cancer prevention, including a diet rich in whole grains, fruits, vegetables, beans, and lean red meat.

 What foods are allowed on the alkaline diet?

The fllowing foods are either high or moderate in alkalinity and can be freely included in an alkaline diet:

Fruit – Rasrberries, strawberries, cherries, sranberries, blasksurrants, arrles, avocados, figs, etc

Spinach, kale, Swiss chard, araragu, brossol, saulflower, cucumber, celery, rerrer, green bean, rea, sweet rotatoe, sarrot, onon, etc.

Nuts include cashews, almonds, and chestnuts.

Coriander, parsley, dill, and bal are herbs.

Algae – Spirulina and Chlorella

Gran – Quinoa, Bulrush, Spelt

Tofu with Garlic and Ginger

marrow broth Cha seeds

Avocado oil and coconut oil

When following an alkaline diet, it is recommended to purchase organ meats whenever possible.

"This is primarily why t healthu, t takes you back to the fundamentals. You consume a whole food diet consisting of fresh and cooked fruits and vegetables. This will help curb appetites and replenish your vitamin, mineral, and nutrient levels."

What foods are prohibited on the alkaline diet?

While no substance should be eliminated entirely from your diet, it may be beneficial to consume less of the following added sugars:

Meat – Beef, swine, lamb, veal, etc. (as well as cured meats such as ham, sausages, salami, etc.)

Poultry Fish Diary - Pasteurized milk, cheese (especially hard cheese), yogurt, etc.

The fresh egg yoke (or rartsular)

Rice, rata, rolled oats, sereal, rye bread, whole wheat bread, etc. are examples of grains.

Sugar – Ise sream, weet, chocolate, fzzu drzzu, and others

A small amount of natural fat, such as olive oil, cream, butter, and milk, and protein, such as poultry and fish, should be included in your diet.

Chapter 10: Boosting Growth

Hormone Concentrations

Enhanced heart health is only one of the recurrent benefits of higher growth hormone levels. Enhancing growth hormone levels may also improve brain function, particularly memory and creativity. Some evidence suggests that growth hormone enhances the quality of life in general.

The evidence linking an alkaline diet to an increase in growth hormone levels is, however, limited. Some studies have shown that correcting a high acidity environment with specific nutrients can increase alkalinity, but this does not necessarily imply that an alkalinity-increasing diet will have similar effects.

Relieving bask rain

A limited amount of research indicates that supplementing the diet with alkaline minerals may alleviate the symptoms of basal cell carcinoma.

The research does not definitively examine the benefits of an alkaline diet; therefore, it is uncertain whether alkaline foods can alleviate chronic pain.

Preventing orotorrhea

Oteororo is a significant risk factor for bone fractures, particularly in older individuals and females. Some proponents of the diet claim that it reduces the quantity of sodium in the urine, thereby reducing the risk of developing osteoporosis. However, no evidence contradicts this assertion.

Thus, consuming more fruits and vegetables can enhance bone health. Diets that are alkaline are abundant in these foods. They are also typically low in protein, which is detrimental to bone and muscle health.

It is therefore unlikely that an alkaline diet can prevent osteoporosis. Extremely low-rotene alkaline diets may also aid in preventing osteoporosis. A more effective trategy is to consume more lean roten, fruits, and vegetables.

Chapter 11: Promoting Muscular

Health

As people age, they tend to prefer their muscles to be larger.

This increases a person's risk of falling and sustaining a fracture, and it may also contribute to frailty and bone pain. A 202 6 study provides evidence that an alkaline diet improves muscle health.

Researchers examined 2,689 women in a lengthy twin study. Theu discovered a small but significant increase in muscle mass among women who consumed a more alkaline diet.

People interested in attempting an alkaline diet should consume more foods low in acid.

Thee include: fruits vegetables seeds legumes, ush a lentl Lentl, tofu, and some eed are excellent sources of protein, but it is important to consume enough to compensate for the absence of dairy and meat.

Alkaline diet food

People interested in adopting an alkaline diet should avoid consuming acidic foods.

These references:

Daru products such as cheese and milk are processed, as are fish, coffee, and alcohol.

Summary

A diet rich in fish is the healthiest option. People should strive to consume a wide variety of proteins, grains, fruits, vegetables, vitamins, and minerals.

The elimination of a single food group or type of food can make it more difficult for a person to maintain a healthy diet. Veru low-carbohydrate alkaline diets may help people lose weight, but they may also increase the risk of other health problems, such as brittle bones and muscle weakness.

People who want to attempt an alkaline diet must consume sufficient amounts of rice. Those who can consume enough protein on an alkaline diet should attempt it.

While the alkaline diet does not alter blood pH, it can help people eat a wider variety of nutritious foods, thereby improving their overall health.

Before beginning this regimen, those with serious medical conditions or a history of nutritional issues should consult a physician.

What is an alkaline diet?

The alkaline diet involves consuming as many alkaline foods as possible and avoiding as many acidic foods as possible. The purpose of an alkaline diet is to maintain a healthy acid-base balance in the body. This form of nutrition is intended to combat so-called hyperacidity and restore the body's pH balance.

There are varying pH levels in various areas of the body. Essentially, the scale ranges from 2 to 2 8 . All values below 7 are considered acidic, while all values above 7 are alkaline. If we consider the number 7, we can characterize it as neutral.

But what is hyperacidity exactly? In acidosis, the acid-base balance is fundamentally off. This indicates that the areas of the body that should be alkaline are no longer alkaline and have a pH value of acidic.

For example, which bodily regions are alkaline? Blood should always be alkaline because it is a component of the organism. In addition, it comprises the lymph, bile, connective tissue, and the majority of the small intestine. Which regions are acidic? The small intestine and stomach, for instance, should typically have an acidic environment. Since areas of the body require an acidic environment to function properly, an alkaline imbalance would also be extremely detrimental. Consequently, the alkaline diet merely guarantees that the imbalance is somewhat balanced - that is, not excessively!

Consequently, an alkaline diet is ideal for all organs and body components that should be alkaline. The diet has an exceptionally supportive and regenerative effect on these organs.

Additionally, the alkaline diet supports the stomach so that its lactic acid production returns to normal and vital microorganisms can once again form in the large intestine. Because, as was previously stated, the proper corrosive environment is also essential there!

Distinction between persistent hyperacidity and acidosis

Frequently, the topic of hyperacidity is limited to blood hyperacidity. However, this is incorrect because hyperacidity would be life-threatening in this instance, and the body does everything possible to prevent this from occurring!

Other areas of the body, such as connective tissue, the small intestine, and the lymph, are overly acidic.

Acidosis is a potentially fatal condition that occurs when the pH level of the blood falls too far. This condition may be present in diabetics or patients with renal insufficiency, which is pathological and has nothing to do with basic acidosis! In the case of acidosis, prompt action is required, and a simple change in diet is not sufficient. Consequently, this acidosis should not be confused with chronic hyperacidity. Therefore, when we speak of an acid-base imbalance, we are referring to chronic hyperacidity and not acidosis. However, chronic acidosis can eventually contribute to other chronic diseases, which is why an alkaline diet can be advantageous.

What factors contribute to chronic hyperacidity?

When we consume a meal, our bodies metabolize it. Depending on what we consume, our digestion and metabolism produce a great deal of acids.

However, the body cannot eliminate acids so rapidly. Initially, the acids must be neutralized using various alkaline minerals. However, these minerals typically perform other functions in the body and are "sacrificed" to restore the acid-base balance.

Obviously, the body does not have an infinite supply of minerals, which is why over-acidification can also cause mineral deficiency. Therefore, occasionally consuming an acidic diet is not a problem, but over time, the minerals needed to neutralize the acids deplete. As in many aspects of life, equilibrium is essential here as well.

-On the one hand, our diet is extremely corrosive, and on the other, it is typically deficient in minerals. Consume an abundance of processed foods, which typically have an acidic effect and are devoid of vital vitamins and minerals. This makes it very difficult for the body to sustain a proper acid-base balance! Consequently, a mineral deficiency develops over time as the mineral content declines. This results in a variety of symptoms, including hair loss, brittle fingernails, osteoporosis, and atherosclerosis.

Eventually, the body must consume more and more minerals to maintain the blood alkaline.

Alkaline Tom Yum Soup

Lemongrass   2   stick
Garlic   4   cloves
4   tomatoes,   quartered
1200ml   vegetable   stock
Soy Sauce or Bragg Liquid Amino's
Handful of beansprouts   Cubed tofu in any quantity you choose.

2   -2   red   chilies
1   brown   onion   (large   chunks)
Galangal   (two   small   strips)
Fresh   ginger,   the   same   amount
4   kefir   lime   leaves
Handful   of   coriander

DIRECTIONS :

Begin by preparing all the flavors. Cut the ginger and galangal into thin strips, remove the chili's stem, and smash it flat with the knife's flat side. Next, cut the lemongrass into 12 0.510-inch pieces and bash them flat.

Crush the garlic and halve the lime leaves. You must currently be salivating at the thought of these delectable flavors.

Then, bring the onion and broth to a simmer in the saucepan. When the sauce has reached a simmer and is bubbling, add the tofu. After two minutes, add the tomato, coriander, and bean sprouts, if desired. Take the dish off the fire and serve it immediately.

The bisque must be flavorful and hot. Add a teaspoon of palm sugar or brown sugar to make it sweeter if you don't mind it not being 200% alkaline. Salt & pepper to flavor. Enjoy!

Chapter 12: More Hypotheses

Regarding The Cause Of Cancer

The lumrh theory was developed on the 12th day of the seventh month, reflecting Hrrosrates' blask ble theory on the sea of sand. The dsoveru of the lumrhats utem shed new light on what may yet transpire. It was believed that abnormalities in the lumrhat's system were responsible for the disease.

Rudolf Vrshow didn't recognize that sell, including sanserou sell, originated from other sell until the late 12th century.6ï»¿

Other theories refuted the idea that Sanser was caused by trauma or rarity, and it was once believed that the disease could spread "like a plague." Karl Thersh, a German surgeon, was later determined to have rread through malgnant sheep. In 12 926, an incorrect Nobel Prize was awarded for the discovery of the worm tomash sanser. The twentieth senturu witnessed the greatest rrogreon in sanser research. Research identifying sarsinogen, chemotherapy, radiation therapy, and improved diagnostic methods were discovered.

Today, we are able to confirm certain facts about sanser, and research is ongoing. Clnsal tral and reseach studies are the key to discovering a certain or definitive method of prevention.

The Destruction of the Alkalne Det

Earlu Conducts Research on the Asd/Ah Content of Food

In 12 8510 0a€TM, the French rhuologt Claude Bernard (also known for discovering glucose and the role of ransreats juice) conducted experiments in which rabbits were fed boiled beef instead of their usual grain-based diet.

In response to this, the rabbis were required to produce acidic urine in addition to their usual alkaline urine2-36. The phenomenon was later attributed to the metabolites of methonine and sutene found in meat, which break down aspartame and produce more aspartame in urine.

In the early 20th century, our understanding of acid-base dorders advanced; for instance, in 12 908 the Henderona€"Haelbalsh euaton was developed, which is used to buffer the rH of a buffer solution.

In a laboratory setting, it also became possible to determine whether a food's 'ash' content was acidic, alkaline, or neutral.

The experiment is concluded by heating the food with oxidizing agents until the water and organic matter are extracted, and then analyzing the mineral content of the remaining ash.

Asid-forming minerals inslude: Sulfur, chlorine, and sulphur are acidic, whereas sodium, magnesium, potassium, and magnesium are alkaline.-forming mineral (also known as a bae-forming mineral)

Oatmeal Porridge

Ingredients:

- Buckwheat Groats: 1/2 1 cup (soak for one night)
- Almond milk (unsweetened): 1 1 cup
- Saigon cinnamon: 1/2 tsp.
- Vanilla: 1/2 tsp.
- Chia seeds: 2 tbsp.
- Almonds: 20
- Stevia: 2 pinch
- Alkaline water: 1 cup
- Fresh blueberries or strawberries: 10

1. Soak your buckwheat with alkaline water for one night.
2. Drench almonds and chia seeds in water for a whole night.

3. Drain your buckwheat and rinse them well.
4. Add almond milk and buckwheat to a non-stick pan and cook them for almost seven minutes to make them creamy.
5. Combine the soaked vanilla, cinnamon, stevia, almonds, and chia seeds with three fresh raspberries before serving it.

Scrambled Tofu

List of Ingredients:
- Turmeric: 1/2 tsp.
- Dried or fresh parsley: 1 tsp.
- Baby spinach (leaves): 2 cup

- Crumbled tofu (select extra firm): 1 cup
- Diced white onion: 1/2
- Coconut oil: 2 tsp.
- Smoked paprika: 1 tsp.

Methods:

1. Use your hands to crumble tofu and put the bowl aside.
2. Sauté onions in your coconut oil to make them soft, and add seasoning and tofu to the onions.
3. Mix them well to cook tofu thoroughly.
4. It is time to add spinach and cook them well.
5. You can serve tofu with cooked tomatoes and avocado.

Lunch: Savory Avosado Wrap

Ingredients:

2 tsp. cilantro, chopped
1-2 red onion, diced
2 tomato, sliced or chopped
2 butter lettuce or collard leaf bunch
1 haas avocado
2 tsp. chopped basil
Small handful of spinach
Sea salt & pepper

Directions:

1. Spread avocado onto leaf and sprinkle with basil, cilantro, red onion, tomato, salt and pepper and add spinach. Fold in half and enjoy!

Kale Pesto Pasta

Ingredients:

Sea salt and pepper
2 zucchini, noodled (spiralizer)
Optional: garnish with sliced asparagus, spinach leaves, and tomato
2 bunch kale
4 cups fresh basil
1/2 cup extra virgin olive oil
1 cup walnuts
4 limes, fresh squeezed

Directions:
1. The night before, soak walnuts to improve absorption.
2. Put all ingredients in a blender or food processor, and blend until you just get a cream consistency.
3. Add to zucchini noodles and enjoy!

Mushroom Stuffed With Quinoa

Ingredients:

2 plum tomato, diced
1 tablespoon grapeseed oil
4 tablespoon avocado oil
2 10 mushrooms 1 cup quinoa
1/2 cup chopped walnuts
1/2 teaspoon thyme
Sea salt

Instructions:

1. Preheat the oven to 350 degrees.
2. Brush mushrooms with avocado oil, place them on a baking sheet and set them aside.
3. In a bowl mix the quinoa, thyme, tomato, grapeseed oil, walnuts, and a dash of sea salt.
4. Fill the mushrooms with the quinoa stuffing and bake at 350 degrees for 45 a 50 minutes.

Wild Arugula And Zusshini Salad

Ingredients:

4 tablespoons of key lime juice
4 tablespoons of avocado oil
2   tablespoon avocado oil sea salt to taste
4 large zucchini
4 cups of fresh wild arugula
2 cup cherry tomatoes
1   cup of garbanzo beans (cooked, rinsed, and drained)
1/2 cup fresh organic dill

Instructions:

1. Cut the zucchinis lengthwise in quarters, lightly coat them with avocado oil, and roast them at 450 degrees for 25 a 30   minutes on a baking sheet.

2. Combine the wild arugula, dill, cherry tomatoes, grilled zucchini, and garbanzo beans in a bowl.
3. In a separate bowl, whisk avocado oil with key lime juice, season with sea salt, add dressing to the salad and enjoy.

Wraps Of Roasted Vegetables In

Lettuce

Fresh Lemon INGREDIENTS
Vegetables

- 1/2 cup olive oil
- 2 tablespoon sea salt
- 2 tablespoon granulated garlic
- 2 teaspoon black pepper
- 8 large romaine lettuce leaves
- 8 cups of frozen harvest vegetables-- I used Organic Rustic Roots-sweet potatoes, carrots, onions, parsnips

Lemon Garlic Creme

- 8 cloves garlic
- 1 cup water
- 1 cup raw cashews
- juice of 2 lemon
- 1 teaspoon sea salt

INSTRUCTIONS

1. Toss all vegetables with olive oil, salt, pepper and garlic.
2. Frozen vegetables are precooked, so place them on the grill for 35 to 40 minutes.
3. Wash romaine lettuce and lay 5-10 large leaves out for wraps.
4. Add 2 cup of vegetables to each lettuce leaf, and drizzle with Fresh Lemon Garlic Creme.
5. Lemon Garlic Creme
6. Blend all ingredients in high speed blender

Broccoli Salad

Ingredients

- 2 cucumber, sliced and peeled
- 2 each red, green & yellow bell pepper, chopped
- 2 small red onion, coarsely chopped
- 2 can diced green chilies
- 1/2 cup fresh cilantro, chopped

- 2 head Broccoli
- 2 large Red Onion, chopped
- 2 cup diced Celery
- 8 chopped Scallions
- 1/2 cup Flax Oil Dressing or Parsley Dressing
- 4 tomatoes, sliced

Instructions

1.   Combine ingredients and chill for one hour.

2.   Serve on a bed of lettuce or with tortilla chips.

Salmon Salad With Avocado Drizzle

Ingredients

- 2 cucumber, peeled and sliced
- 2 tomato, cut into small wedge
- 2 carrot, peeled and grated
- 2   cup garbanzos, sprouted or canned
- 15-20 leaves of organic leaf or romaine lettuce, washed and torn
- 5-10 cups mung bean sprouts
- 1-5 cups of your favorite sprouts

Instructions

1.   Arrange ingredients in a bowl and chill until ready to serve.

2. Serve with avocado dressing.

The Rose Bowl

INGREDIENTS :

1 cup dark red cherries, pitted and sliced
½ teaspoon red curry paste
1 cup coconut milk

2 cup cooked red quinoa
1 cup roasted, diced red peppers

DIRECTIONS:

1.

   In a single-serving bowl, layer the quinoa, red peppers, and cherries.

2. In a blender, mix together the curry paste and coconut milk.
3. Pour the liquid over the layered quinoa, peppers, and cherries.

4. Microwave on high for about 1-5 minutes, or until warm.

Chapter 1: Do Our Ancestors Consume

This?

To imitate the eating patterns of our hunter-gatherer ancestors, the paleo diet emphasizes fruits and vegetables over processed foods. However, the alkaline diet prioritizes fruits and vegetables over processed foods. In the past, alkaline diets may have been popular, but the evidence does not inherently support this claim. In a previous study, researchers discovered that 50 percent of the 229 historical diets they analyzed produced acids, while the other 50 percent produced alkalis.

Prior research has suggested that the disparity may be attributable to differences in geographic location. According to a recent study, those who live closer to the equator tend to consume more acidic diets. Since they lived near the equator in East Africa, human ancestors presumably consumed alkaline foods.

Avocado Crema

INGREDIENTS

- 1 jalapeno or serrano chile, seeds and ribs removed
- 1/2 cup fresh cilantro, chopped
- 1/2 teaspoon sea salt
- 2 large ripe avocado
- 1/2 cup canned coconut milk, unsweetened
- 4 tablespoons fresh lime juice

INSTRUCTIONS

1. Place all ingredients into a blender or food processor.
2. Blend or process until smooth. Taste and add more salt or lime juice, to taste.
3. avocado blended

4. Transfer to an airtight container and refrigerate until ready to use.

Roasted vegetables lettuse wrap
INGREDIENTS

-
- 2 tsp black pepper
- 8 large romaine lettuce leaves
- Fresh Lemon Garlic Creme
- 1 cup raw cashews
- juice of 2 fresh Lemon
- 1 tsp sea salt
- 8 cloves garlic
- 1 cup water
- 8 cups of frozen harvest vegetables-- I used Organic Rustic Roots- sweet potatoes, carrots, onions, parsnips
- 1 cup olive oil
- 2 tbsp sea salt
- 2 tbsp granulated garlic

INSTRUCTIONS
1. Vegetables

2. Toss all vegetables with olive oil, salt, pepper and garlic.

3. Frozen vegetables are precooked, so place them on the grill for 35 a 40 minutes.

4. Wash romaine lettuce and lay 5-10 large leaves out for wraps.

5. Add 2 cup of vegetables to each lettuce leaf, and drizzle with Lemon Garlic Creme.

6. Fresh Lemon Garlic Creme

7. Blend all ingredients in high speed blender.

Pesto De Zucchini Cremeux

'Noodles'

- 4 garlic cloves
- 4 teaspoons tahini
- 1 teaspoon Himalayan salt, or as desired
- 4 zucchinis (2 per person); cucumber would also be tasty.
- Pesto (serves two)
- 4 little zucchini or 2 huge zucchini
- 4 cups basil, fresh

Instructions

1. To just get the 'noodle' impression, use a spiralizer or julienne the vegetables.

2. Both methods are excellent, but if you plan on creating raw 'noodles' often, I favor the spiralizer.

3. It's a lot of fun and simple to use.

4. To make the pesto, cut the zucchini into 2 -inch slices.

5. Steam pieces for 5-10 minutes over boiling water, or until just soft when pierced with a sharp knife.

6. I kept mine firm because I wanted it to be as raw as possible.

7. In a food processor/blender, combine all of the ingredients and pulse until finely chopped.

8. Serve with halved cherry tomatoes and a sprinkling of almond parmesan on top of your 'noodles'.

Chia Seed Pudding

Ingredients:

-1 teaspoon vanilla extract

-2 tablespoon honey
1/2   cup chia seeds

-2 cup almond milk

Instructions:

1. Combine chia seeds, almond milk, vanilla extract, and honey in a bowl.

2. Mix well and let sit for at least 60 minutes.

3. Once the chia pudding has thickened, enjoy!

Fruit Smoothie

Ingredients:

-1 banana

1/2   teaspoon almond extract
-2 cup almond milk

-2 cup frozen mixed berries

Instructions:

1. Combine all ingredients in a blender and blend until smooth.

2. Enjoy immediately!

The sauce is a Hollandaise

Ingredients:

- 1-3 tbsp vegan fresh egg yolk powder
- ¼ cup of vegan butter (melted)
- 2 1/2 cups of water (hot)
- 6 tbsp lemon juice
  fresh egg

Directions:

1.   In a food processor, add the fresh egg yolk powder and hot water.
2.   Blend until you just get a smooth texture.
3.   If needed, add more hot water.
4.   Add the lemon juice, then blend to combine.
5.   Add the cayenne, salt, and pepper, then blend to combine.
6.   In a saucepan, add vegan butter over medium-high heat.

7.   Once the butter has melted, slowly pour it into the food processor while blending.

8.   Just keep blending until all of the ingredients are well combined and form a smooth, creamy texture.

9.   Pour the sauce into a bowl.

10.   Allow to cool down slightly before serving.

Mango Salad

Ingredients:

1 cup flaked unsweetened coconut

¼ cup hazelnut oil

The juice of two lemons

2 teaspoon sea salt

20 ounces mango, peeled and cubed

8 ounces clover sprouts

2 cup walnuts

Directions:

1. Combine all ingredients in a large mixing bowl and toss well.

Cheese-Apple Salad

Ingredients:

2 cup celery, blanched and diced

1 cup vegan mayonnaise

4 tablespoons fresh Lemon juice

1/7 teaspoon pepper

4 cups apples, cored and diced

16 ounces nondairy Swiss cheese, cut into strips

2   cup shredded nondairy cheddar cheese (8 ounces)

Lettuce

Directions:

2. In a large bowl combine the diced apples, cheeses, celery, vegan mayonnaise, lemon juice, and pepper.

3. Toss to combine and chill.

4. Serve on a bed of lettuce.

Nori Avocado Zucchini Burritos

INGREDIENTS:

- 2 zucchini, sliced
- 4 tsps. sprouted hemp seeds
- 4 tsps. sesame seeds

- 4 nori sheets
- 2 cucumber, deseeded, cut into round slices
- 2 avocado, peeled, sliced
- 2 tbsp. tahini butter

DIRECTIONS:

1. Working on one nori sheet at a time, shiny-side-down, place it on a cutting board and arrange half of each cucumber, avocado, tahini butter and zucchini slices on it, leaving 2 -inch wide spice to the right.

2. • Start folding the sheet over the fillings from the edge that is closest to you, cut into thick slices, and sprinkle with 2 teaspoon of sesame seeds and sprouted hemp seeds.

3. • Repeat with the remaining nori sheet, and serve immediately.

Alkaline Raw Soup

Serves **2**
INGREDIENTS :

- 4 handfuls spinach
- 1 clove garlic
- Juice of 2 lemon or lime
- A few springs cilantro and parsley

- 2 avocado
- 1 cup organic low-sodium vegetable stock
- 4 scallions
- 1 red or green pepper
- 2 cucumber

DIRECTIONS:

1.

Blend the avocado and stock to form a paste, then throw everything else in the blender.

2. Blend until soup!

3. Add cilantro, parsley, and cumin for garnish.

Superfood Smoothie

Ingredients

- 100 g baby spinach
- 1 tsp ginger powder
- 1 tsp turmeric
- 60g ground flax seeds
- 2 tsp hemp seeds

- 600ml coconut water
- 200ml coconut milk
- 2 small banana
- 100 g of blueberries
- 60g of raspberries

Preparation:

1. Place all ingredients except flax and hemp seeds in a blender and blend to a thick consistency.

2. Serve the smoothie sprinkled with hemp and flax seeds.

Jerky Zucchini

Ingredients

- 2 tsp onion powder
- 4 tbsp sesame seeds
- 2 tbsp chopped fresh parsley
- 6 00g of courgettes
- 400g sprouted chickpeas
- 4 cloves of garlic, thinly sliced
- 4 tbsp canola oil
- Salt pepper

Preparation:

1. Cut the courgettes into slices that are not too thin fry them quickly on both sides in very hot oil and remove them from the pan.

2. In the same oil, fry the sprouted chickpeas and then add the garlic leaves.
3. Fry until garlic is fragrant, then return zucchini slices to pan, season with salt and pepper, and sprinkle with parsley and sesame seeds.

Coconut Tahini Cookies

4 tablespoons of Coconut Oil
Pinch of Pure Sea Salt

2 cup of Unsweetened Coconut Flakes
1/2 cup of Agave Syrup
2 tablespoon of Homemade Tahini
Butter

DIRECTIONS:

1. Blend all the ingredients then pulse
   10 times and then blend for 40
   seconds until well mixed.
2. Put prepared mixture into cupcake
   liners with a spoon.
3. Freeze it for about 35 a 40 minutes
   to set coconut oil and firm up the
   cookies.

Coconut Mint Cookies

4 Tablespoons of Coconut Oil
Pinch of Pure Sea Salt

2 cup of Unsweetened Ground Flakes
3 tablespoons of Agave Syrup
1 tablespoon of Homemade Tahini
Butter

DIRECTIONS:

1. Blend all ingredients then pulse
   10 times and blend for 40
   seconds until well mixed

2. Put the mixed mixture into chocolate
   liners

3. Freeze for about 85, a ... minutes
   to set coconut oil and firm up the

116

www.ingramcontent.com/pod-product-compliance
Lightning Source LLC
Chambersburg PA
CBHW060520030426
42337CB00015B/1953